# 20 Awesome Raw Dinners Recipes You Can't Live Without

# Raw Food Recipes for a Healthy Lifestyle

## By Kathy Tennefoss

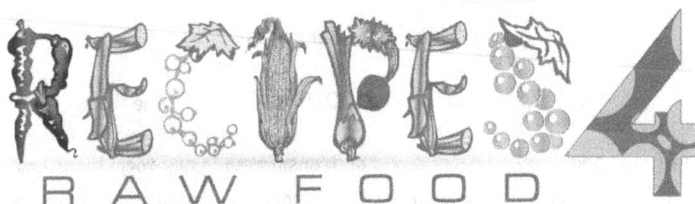

RECIPES 4
RAW FOOD

## Member of the Raw Foods Association

# RECIPES 4
## RAW FOOD

**20 Awesome Raw Dinners You Can't Live Without**

**Sunny Cabana Publishing, L.L.C.**

**Fort Lauderdale, FL**

www.sunnycabanapublishing.com

By Kathy Tennefoss

Published by Kathleen Tennefoss
Printed in the United States of America
Author: Kathy Tennefoss
Editor: Shawn M Tennefoss
13-digit ISBN: 9781936874071
10-digit ISBN: 1936874075
SECOND EDITION
Library of Congress Cataloging-in-Publication Data has been applied for

This book is dedicated to My dad James Kelley for pushing me in the right direction regarding health food and living a healthy life and to my loving husband Shawn Tennefoss for putting up with my computer difficulties and taking the time to show me how to facilitate my publishing efforts along with sharing his life and journey with me.

Cover Design: Kathy & Shawn Tennefoss

Second Edition, 2011

Acknowledgements:

Thanks to everyone who encouraged and inspired me and gave me great ideas and feedback in the raw food industry, including one of my many sisters Heather McNerney, my husband Shawn m Tennefoss, my dad James Kelley, and Melissa Hernandez and her wonderful family! Without everyone's input I would not have finished this or other raw food recipe books that I have in the works! I am extremely grateful to everyone!

**Disclaimer:**

The responsibility for any adverse detoxification effects resulting from using these recipes described lies not with the author or distributors of this book. This book is not intended for medical advice just as suggestion.

Please enjoy these recipes with your families!

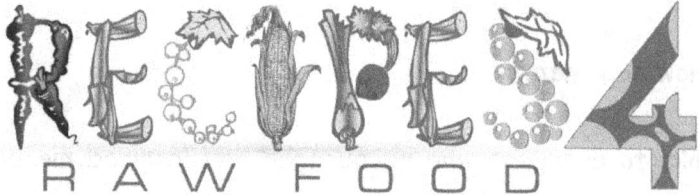

# Introduction

In this book *20 Awesome Raw Main Dishes You Can't Live With-out.* I have gone through only some of my recipes that I found are the easiest to make when you are short on time. Everyone is busy but you still should make the time to eat a healthy meal for you and your family. It's also about putting fun into your meals by involving the whole family and have them help and give their input so that they feel like they are contributing to their own health because when your children get older they will remember this and pass the healthy living on to their children. I know this from experience. I had a father who ate healthy mostly vegetarian meals and biked and a mother who ate only junk food and did not exercise whatsoever.  It was a battle at our house of what to eat. I never knew who to go with but at least I had the option and that is why I feel so compelled to tell others about healthy eating.

I didn't realize until I got older how my father influenced me and my food choices.  My mother was always sick and did not take care of herself very well and that was to her detriment. I vowed to myself and my family that I would try my hardest to seek out the best quality food by purchasing organic produce and by preparing the food as to not lose its nutritional value and I have stuck to that promise for over 20 years. I feel that this has helped me and my family immensely and I want to pass the benefits on to others so that they too will feel that they are contributing to a better way of life!

Please try all of my recipes and put your best foot forward in the fight for obesity, diabetes, heart disease, cancer, and a slew of other ailments that are from not eating a healthy diet. Also remember that life should be fun and that eating healthy doesn't mean that you have to be strict every single day. It's the small efforts that you put forth everyday that make a difference in the long run! People will start to notice your healthy glow and how young you look and start to ask you how, what, and will you show me. This is when you will feel like you have made a difference in the world.

# Table of Contents

## Collard Wraps

6 Medium Collard Leaves (washed with the stem taken off if they are too long)

1 Cup Shredded Carrots

1 Cup 1 inch thinly sliced Cucumbers

1 Cup Thinly Sliced Red Peppers

1 Cup Sprouts

$\frac{1}{4}$ Cup Raw Sunflower Seeds

$\frac{1}{2}$ Cup of some type of spread like raw pesto, raw sundried tomato spread, hummus

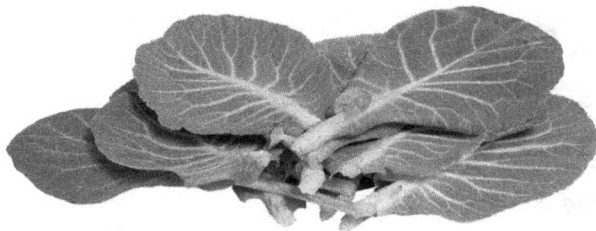

(whatever one you like the best)

Take the washed collard greens and lay them flat. First put the spread of your choice in the middle of the leaf then put some of each of the rest of the ingredients and wrap like a burrito! Yum these are so good and good for you too!

**Crunchy Lettuce Wraps**

A Small head of Bib Lettuce or Romaine (cleaned and washed)

1 Cup Jicama (peeled and sliced into thin 1 inch pieces)

$\frac{1}{2}$ Cup Cilantro cleaned (not chopped; just kept in single strands)

1 Cup thinly sliced Red Peppers

2 Cup of Bean Sprouts

1/2 Cup Chopped Raw Peanuts (for top)

$\frac{1}{2}$ Cup Lime Peanut sauce (this is a simple sauce of raw peanut butter mixed with Lime juice to the consistency of a thin sauce)

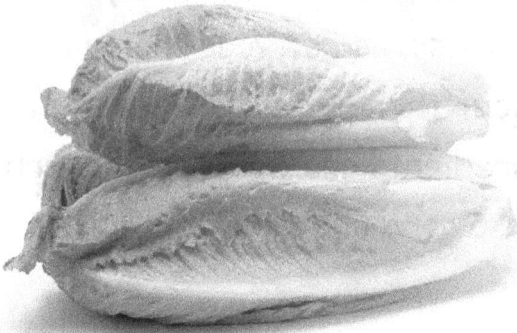

Take the Bib Lettuce or Romaine (I like Bib because it is a little softer and easier to handle when you are eating it) and put some of each ingredient inside and wrap it up and serve with either the peanut sauce or put the peanut sauce inside the wrap.  I like it with both!

**Sweet Nori Wraps**

> 1 Cup Strawberries thinly sliced
> 1 Cup Papaya Thinly Sliced
> 1 Cup Mango Thinly Sliced

$\frac{1}{4}$ Cup Mint Leaves Whole

Cashew Dipping Sauce, which is 1 cup cashews soaked for 4 hours and then drained. Put the soaked cashews into a vitamixer along with 2 Tablespoons of lime juice, and 1 tablespoon of agave nectar, and a small amount of water or $\frac{1}{2}$ an orange squeezed to make the right consistency for a sauce.

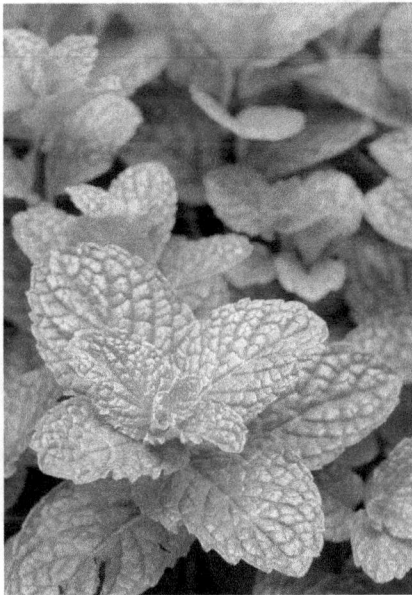

Keep the nori sheets dry on a cutting board and start to fill the nori at the end that is closest to you with the fruits and then start rolling the nori up. After that you will slice the nori into smaller sushi style pieces and dip the pieces into the dipping sauce.

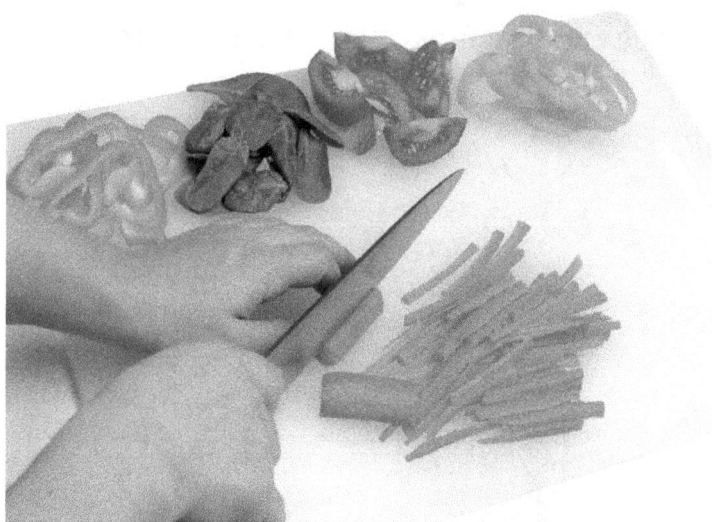

**Veggie Nori Wraps**

1 Cup Thinly sliced Zucchini
1 Cup Thinly Sliced Carrots
1 Cup Thinly Sliced Red Pepper

2 Avocados
1 Cup Thinly Sliced Cucumber
1 cup of Basil Leaves

Take the vegetables and clean and peel them then take the carrot, red pepper, and cucumber and make thin slices the length of the vegetable. Take the avocados and deseed them and mash them up into a spread.

Again keep the nori sheets dry and start and the end closest to you and put a thin layer of the avocado spread on the beginning of the nori sheet, then some of each of the other veggies and then roll it, slice it, and eat it! You can use Braggs for a dipping sauce if you like or whatever you like best.

# Sun Dried Tomato & Arugula Pizza

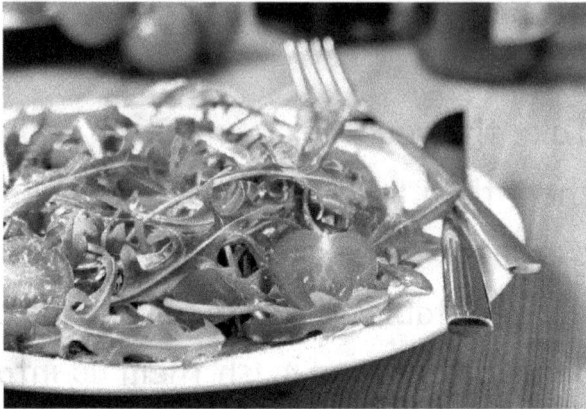

2 Cups of Arugula

1 Cup Sundried Tomato Spread (which is $\frac{3}{4}$ Cup of sundried tomatoes soaked and drained. Using a vitamixer grind up the sundried tomatoes along with $\frac{1}{4}$ cup olive oil, salt and pepper, $\frac{1}{4}$ cup raw pine nuts & half of the basil)

4-5 Seed, Flax, etc Dehydrated crackers of your liking. You can purchase these in most health food stores or if you feel ambitious you can also make them yourself!

$\frac{1}{4}$ Cup basil

Take the flax crackers and spread the sundried tomato spread on the top. Take the arugula and the rest of the basil and mix it with a little balsamic and olive oil (just enough to barely coat the arugula) and then put the arugula on top of the sun dried tomato spread and your done! This is a great treat. You can also use other items like tomatoes sliced, green peppers, red peppers, etc.

# Mushroom & Tomato Pesto Pizza

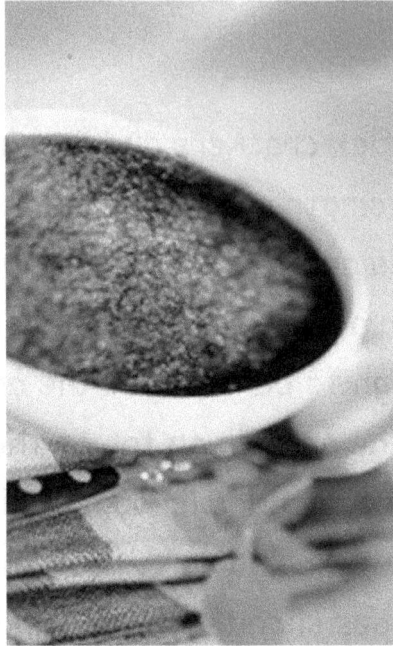

4-5 Flax, Italian, etc dehydrated crackers
Pesto Sauce (1 Cup walnuts soaked for 4-5
hours and drained, 1 Cup basil leaves, $\frac{1}{4}$-1/2
Cup of olive oil, 1/8 cup lime juice 1 clove of
garlic and salt and pepper to taste. Using
the vitamixer grind all of the ingredients
together to a smooth consistency (you may

need a little water or extra olive oil it will just depend).
1 Cup Sliced Tomatoes
1 Cup Sliced Crimini Mushrooms

Take the Italian crackers and spread the raw pesto on the top and then add the sliced tomatoes and mushrooms and sprinkle with basil.


## Mediterranean Burritos


2 Cups Sprouted Garbanzo Beans (see my website www.rawfoodfortoday.com) or soak the beans for 8 hours and allow to sprout for 2-3 days
1/2 Cup Olive Oil
¼ Cup Raw Tahini Butter

6-8 Bib Lettuce leaves not broken

1 Cup Sliced Cucumbers in 1 inch pieces
1 Cup Red Peppers sliced into 1 inch pieces
1 Cup Diced Tomatoes
1 Bunch of Chopped Cilantro
Salt and Pepper

In a food processor combine garbanzo beans, tahini butter, olive oil, and salt and pepper and blend until smooth. Next spread the garbanzo bean mixture on the inside of the bib lettuce and arrange the raw veggies and wrap it up and eat it! This is great because you can put all kinds of veggies in these and change it up a little more.

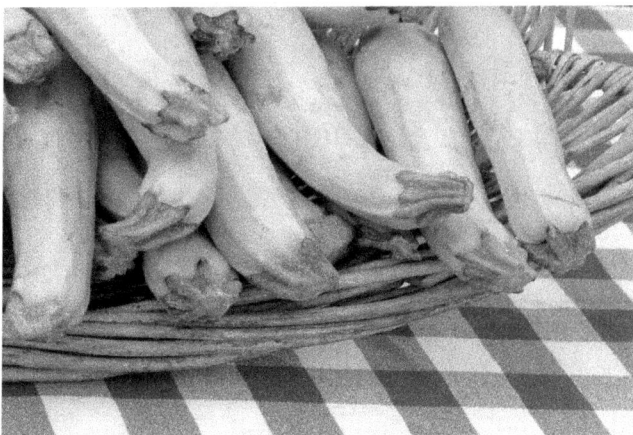

## Alfredo Raw Pasta

3-4 Medium Yellow Zucchini Use a spiral slicer and slice all of the zucchini into long spirals

2 Cups of raw cashews soaked for 4-6 hours
¼ Cup Olive Oil
1 Clove of garlic
½ Cup of Lemon Juice
Salt and Pepper
¼ Cup of Basil
1/8 Cup of Braggs Amino Acids

This is one of my favorite meals! I love this! Once you have the zucchini sliced put it in a large bowl. Now take the soaked cashews and drain them and put the cashews and the rest of the ingredients into a vitamixer and blend until it is a smooth sauce. Next put the sauce on the zucchini and sprinkle with basil.

## Pesto Linguini

3-4 Zucchini or Squash

2 Cups Raw Walnuts Nuts Soaked for 4-6 hours

1 $\frac{1}{2}$ Cups of Basil

$\frac{1}{2}$ Cup Oil

Salt and Pepper

1  Clove of garlic

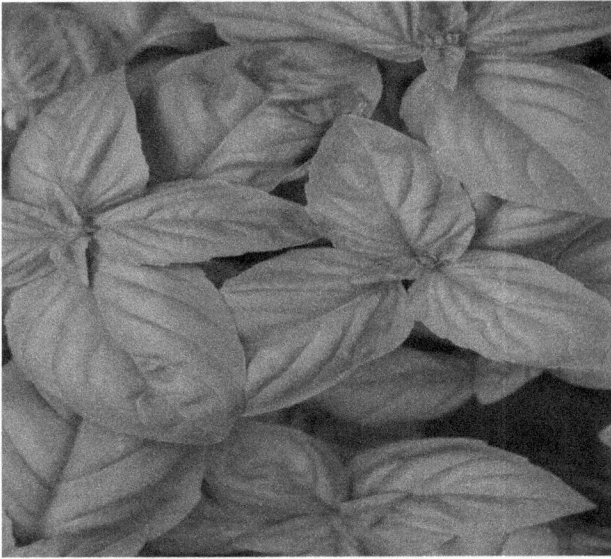

Start with taking the zucchini or squash and cutting it into a large square by cutting the skin off. Then cut that in half and take a peeler and make strips out of both halves so that they look like fettuccini. Then take the walnuts and drain them but save the water in case you need more liquid for the sauce and then add the rest of the ingredients and blend into a sauce. Then take the pesto and toss the zucchini with it and you are done. You can add sliced red peppers if you like to add more color and nutrition.  It's all up to you.

**Spaghetti Squash with Spicy Garlic Sauce**

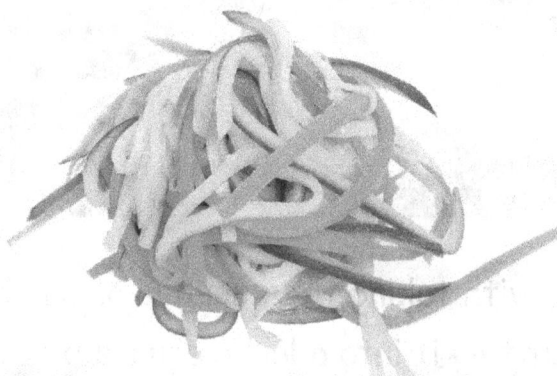

1 Whole Spaghetti Squash

Sliced Carrots

Sliced Green Zucchini

1 Clove of Garlic

½ Cup of Olive Oil

½ teaspoon of red chili peppers

Salt and pepper

This recipe is so easy you will wonder why you don't eat this everyday! First you put the olive oil, chopped garlic, chili peppers, and salt and pepper into a small bowl to blend the flavors. Then you cut the squash in half and then start to scrap the squash out so that there are strings of the squash that look like spaghetti. I use a spoon with sharp points on the end so that it breaks up the squash better. Then you put the squash in a bowl and toss it with the olive oil mixture. If you want you can add slivered red peppers or chopped tomatoes to give the dish more color. If you don't like hot dishes you can also omit the chili peppers. It's really up to your taste buds.

## Italian Caprese Towers

3-4 Large Heirloom Tomatoes

Sliced Onion (whichever kind you like best)
2 Cups Sliced Marinated Portobello's (in a bowl soak the sliced mushrooms in $\frac{1}{2}$ Cup Balsamic vinegar, $\frac{1}{2}$ cup tamari, and $\frac{1}{4}$ cup olive oil for 4-6 hours)

Pesto from recipe number 9
Raw Ricotta

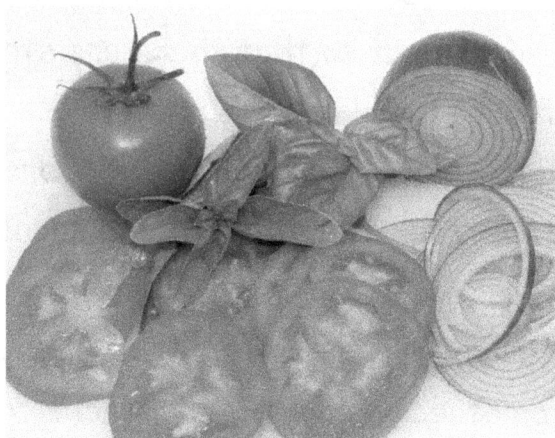

First slice the tomatoes. On a large plate arrange the ingredients in layers starting with the tomatoes, then pesto, then portabellas, then Raw Ricotta (which is 2 cups raw pine nuts, salt and pepper, 3 tablespoons of lemon juice, 1 tablespoon of nutritional yeast, and a couple teaspoons of olive oil. Place all ingredients in a food processor until combined well) and finally the onion. Keep building little towers on the large plate so that everyone gets one or two.

# Lasagna

4-5 Thinly Sliced Zucchini

3-4 Cups Marinated Portobello's (recipe 11)

Raw Ricotta (in Recipe 11)

6-8 Medium Tomatoes

1 Cup Chopped Basil

1 Clove of Garlic

$\frac{1}{4}$ Cup Olive Oil

1 Tablespoon oregano or Italian spices

First start by making the tomato sauce. Using a vitamixer put the tomatoes, basil, garlic, olive oil spices, and salt and pepper and blend until it looks like a nice thick sauce. Now take a glass baking dish and start to layer the thinly sliced zucchini, then ricotta sauce, tomato sauce, and then start another layer using the portabellas mushrooms, ricotta, and then sauce. Keep doing this until all of the ingredients are used up and top with some freshly chopped basil.

## Stuffed Tomatoes

> 7-8 Large Tomatoes
>
> 1 Cup Chopped Basil
>
> 1 Clove Garlic
>
> 1/8 Cup of Olive Oil
>
> Salt and Pepper
>
> 1 Large Jicama peeled
>
> 1 Cup Raw Pine Nuts Soaked for 2 hours

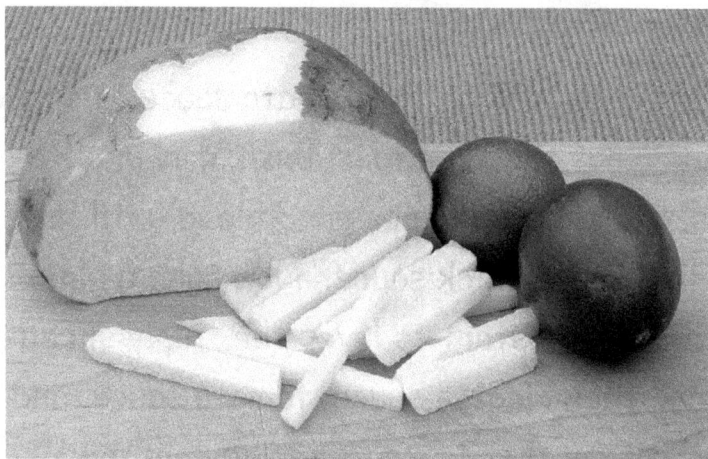

First Take all of the tomatoes and cut into halves. Then scoop out the inside of the tomatoes and then place them in a large glass baking sheet. Next take the rest of the ingredients and blend in a food processor (leaving out $\frac{1}{2}$ cup of the basil for garnish) until smooth and then fill the tomatoes with the filling and top with basil and serve!

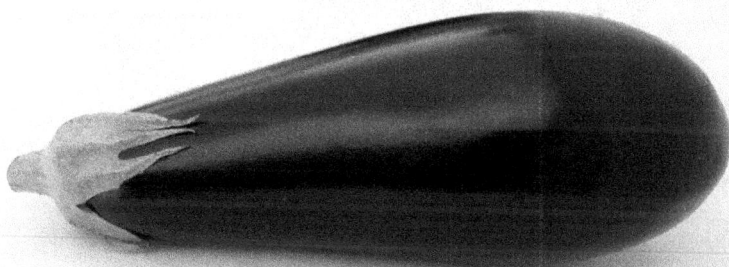

## Ravioli

1 Eggplant sliced into very thin rounds with a mandolin
Raw Ricotta (in recipe 11)
Pesto Sauce (recipe number 9)

Place the thinly sliced eggplant in a bowl of water with 1 tablespoon of salt and let soak for 2 hours, then drain and pat dry. Now add the raw ricotta and fold in half and drizzle with olive oil and pesto sauce. You can use other raw sauces if you would like such as marinara, sun dried tomato, etc.

## Quinoa Summer Salad

1 Cup Sprouted Quinoa (Soak for 2 hours and let sprout for 1 day)
$\frac{1}{4}$ Cup Chopped Mint
1 Cup Cucumber diced into small pieces
1 Cup Red and Green Peppers Chopped into small Pieces
$\frac{1}{2}$ Cup Chopped Parsley
1 Clove of Garlic chopped fine
$\frac{1}{2}$ Cup Olive Oil
$\frac{1}{2}$ Cup Lemon Juice

Salt and Pepper

Mix all ingredients in a bowl and serve.

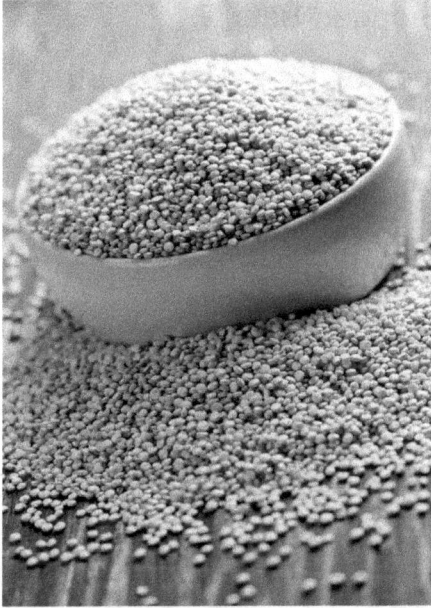

**Thai Wild Rice Salad**

2 Cups Wild Rice soaked for 9 hours and
sprouted for 3-5 days
1 Cup finely chopped Celery
1 Cup Diced Carrots
$\frac{1}{2}$ Cup Diced Red Pepper

1 teaspoon of Ginger

1 Clove of Garlic Chopped Fine

1 Cup Chopped Raw Peanuts

1/2 Cup Chopped Basil

1 Tablespoon of Raw Almond Butter

½ Cup Chopped Cilantro

½-3/4 Cup Lime Juice

¼ Cup Olive Oil

Salt and Pepper

Dash of Chili Peppers

Mix all ingredients together and serve.

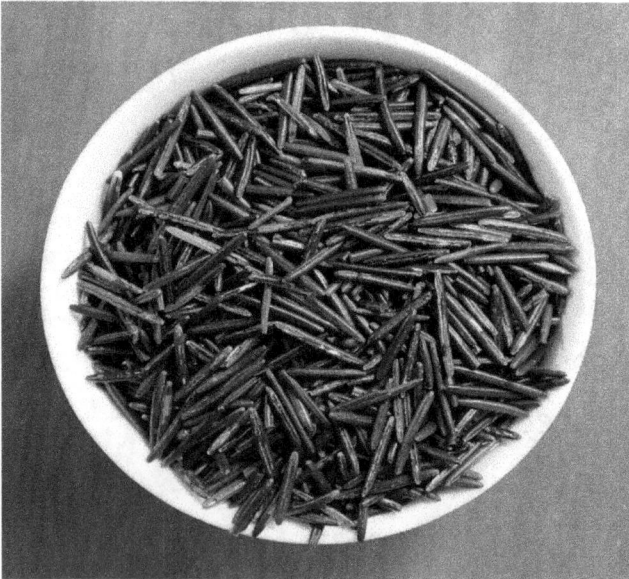

# Sweet Summer Wild Rice Salad

2 Cups Wild Rice soaked for 9 hours and sprouted for 3-5 days

1 Large Red Apple Cut into small pieces

1 Celery Stalk cut into small pieces

1 Cup of Dried Currants

1 Cup Chopped Raw Cashews

$\frac{1}{4}$ Cup Chopped Parsley

1 Tablespoon of Olive Oil

1 Teaspoon of agave nectar

Salt and Pepper

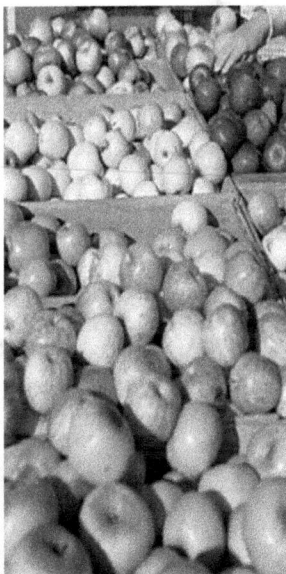

Mix all ingredients in a bowl and serve.

# Raw Burger

- 2 Cups of Raw Walnuts
- 2 Cups carrots
- ¼ Cup Celery
- 1 Clove of garlic
- 1 Shallot
- 1 Teaspoon of agave nectar
- 1 Pitted Date
- 1 Tablespoon of olive oil
- 1 Tablespoon of Italian seasoning
- Salt and Pepper

Mix all ingredients in a food processor until blended. The mixture should be easily shaped into round patties. Then dress with sliced tomatoes, onions, cucumbers, etc.

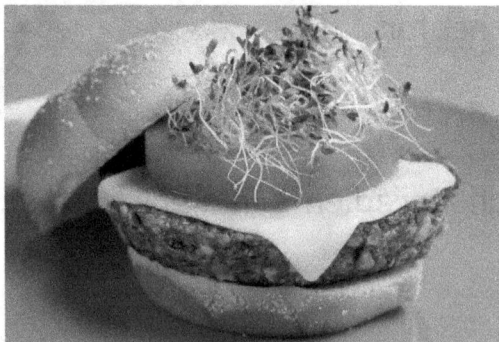

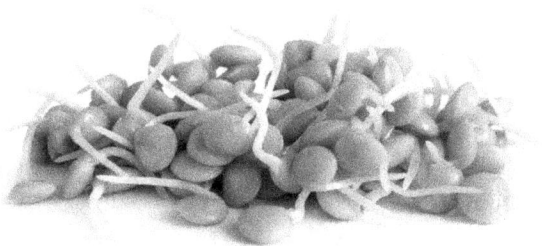

## Lentil Salad

2 Cups lentils soaked for 7 hours and sprouted for 3 days
1/2 Cup Lemon Juice
1 Cup Chopped Parsley
1 Cup Small Diced Tomatoes
$\frac{1}{4}$ Cup Olive Oil
Salt and Pepper
1 Teaspoon of Cumin

Mix all ingredients in a bowl and serve.

## Italian Barley Salad

>  2 Cups Barley soaked for 6 hours and
>  sprouted for 2 days
>  1 Cup Sundried Tomatoes Soaked for 4
>  hours
>  1 Clove of Garlic Chopped fine
>  1 Cup Pitted and Chopped Black Olives
>  $\frac{1}{2}$ Cup Chopped Basil
>  $\frac{1}{4}$-1/2 Cup Olive Oil
>  Salt and Pepper

Drain the sun dried tomatoes and chopped into small pieces. Take the rest of the ingredients and mix in a bowl and serve.

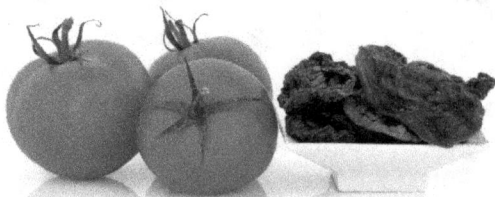

Thanks for taking the time to try these healthy recipes. You will be glad you did. Also I would like to take a minute to tell you how important it is to purchase organic produce.

## Why Eat Organic?

Eating organic is a choice that most of us ponder every day. I know I always chose organic when I can or when I have enough money. But what does organic mean? The first organic produce law was in 1990 from congress and it stated that food grown without pesticides, fungicides, or not genetically modified would be considered organic. Pesticides are toxic and bad for the environment, farmers, and for you and your family. Genetically modified food (food that is made to be larger, better coloring, and pest resistant) has been questioned by many people. No one really knows the long - term effects of this on your body.

Some of the highest levels of pesticide residue on produce that is considered not organic are apricots, nectarines, green beans, potatoes, bananas, cucumbers, celery, corn, peppers, cherries, apples, spinach, tomatoes, soy beans, rice, strawberries, dates, carrots, grapes, peaches, pears, lemons, milk, and sweet potatoes. So I guess if you don't eat any of these your o.k. Well that sounds like a lot of fruits and vegetables to me. There have been numerous studies showing how foods grown without pesticides and fungicides have more nutritional value and a much higher mineral content. Even if the nutritional level was a little better don't you think that you would want that for you and your family? It is also very important to drink organic milk or milk products that have been made without growth hormone and antibiotics. I think I will take my antibiotics from the doctor thank you!

Some ways to get more organic produce in your daily diet is to shop at local farmers markets, ask your local supermarket to carry more organic choices, at the seasonal farmers markets buy extra so you can dehydrate or freeze your extras for the winter months, start a garden, order online and have it delivered, become a member of a food co-op, start a food co-op, or participate in a organic food buying club. These are some simple ways to introduce organic food into you and your family's diet. You and your family are worth it. The more demand in the market place for organic produce the soy beans, rice, strawberries, dates, carrots, grapes, peaches, pears, lemons, milk, and sweet potatoes. So I guess if you don't eat any of these your o.k.

Well that sounds like a lot of fruits and vegetables to me. There have been numerous studies showing how foods grown without pesticides and fungicides have more nutritional value and a much higher mineral content. Even if the nutritional level was a little better don't you think that you would want that for you and your family? It is also very important to drink organic milk or milk products that have been made without growth hormone and antibiotics. I think I will take my antibiotics from the doctor thank you!

Some ways to get more organic produce in your daily diet is to shop at local farmers markets, ask your local supermarket to carry more organic choices, at the seasonal farmers markets buy extra so you can dehydrate or freeze your extras for the winter months, start a garden, order online and have it delivered, become a member of a food co-op, start a food co-op, or participate in a organic food buying club. These are some simple ways to introduce organic food into you and your family's diet. You and your family are worth it. The more demand in the market place for organic produce the cheaper it will eventually be. Do your part in helping the environment and support your local farmers. It only takes a few people in every town to make a difference. Let it be you!

## About the author:

B.S. Science in Physical Anthropology minor in business, and Culinary Arts Degree. Advocate for organic, vegetarian, vegan, raw food diets, writing, yoga, swimming, biking, and running 5 K's!
I have been a vegetarian/vegan/raw foodist for over 20 years. I have also worked in real estate for over ten years and have several websites to help people who are interested in raw food
http://www.Recipes4RawFood.com
http://www.RawFoodForToday.com

I have also started the *Raw Foods Association* with my husband so that others can become members of a larger healthy group and its website is www.RawFoodsAssociation.com !
For more information on how to order books, original articles, become a member of the Raw Foods Association, and updates on future projects go to www.rawfoodfortoday.com or www.recipes4rawfood.com!

Please feel free to email me if you have any comments, suggestions, or corrections to recipes4rawfood@yahoo.com

**Recipes 4 Raw Food**
**1314 E Las Olas Blvd**
**Fort Lauderdale, FL 33301**